Bones, Bodies, and Bellies

Diane A. Vaszily
Peggy K. Perdue

Illustrations by
Karen Waiksnis DiSorbo

Good Year Books
Parsippany, New Jersey

Dedicated to Roberta Dempsey for the inspiration she provided!

Good Year Books
are available for most basic curriculum subjects plus many enrichment areas. For more GoodYearBooks, contact your local bookseller or educational dealer. For a complete catalog with information about other GoodYearBooks, please write:

Good Year Books
An imprint of Pearson Learning
299 Jefferson Road
Parsippany, New Jersey 07054-0480
1-800-321-3106
www.pearsonlearning.com

Book design by Amy O'Brien Krupp.

ISBN 0-673-36034-2

6 7 8 9 - MH - 01 00

Preface

We know that if children are to succeed, they must have positive self-concepts. Teachers across the United States use various techniques to boost self-esteem in their students. We need to take this a step further.

Children in the United States are not physically fit, and this contributes to low self-esteem in many children. Increased television viewing, lack of physical activity, and poor diets are contributing to childhood obesity. It is time to teach our students to take care of themselves. To help do this, we present *Bones, Bodies, and Bellies.*

Bones, Bodies, and Bellies provides the student with opportunities to explore how humans are put together, how the body works, and how to keep it working. Extension activities allow the student to investigate the concepts further.

The style of *Bones, Bodies, and Bellies* is easy to follow. Once familiar with the purpose behind this book and the design of the explorations, you will be able to take ideas, both old and new, and put them into the same framework. Science will no longer be another activity designed to fill the allotted time, but will become relevant to each child in every classroom.

Help your students discover, understand, and take care of the most amazing creatures on earth—themselves!

Contents

Bones

Anatomy—How We're Put Together

From Bones, Bodies and Bellies, published by GoodYearBooks. Copyright © 1994 Diane A. Vaszily and Peggy K. Perdue.

Bodies

Physiology—How We Work

Bellies

Nutrition—Keeping the Body Running

Appendix

From *Bones, Bodies and Bellies*, published by GoodYearBooks. Copyright © 1994 Diane A. Vaszily and Peggy K. Perdue.

How to Use This Book

If you are looking for hands-on, relevant science activities for a unit on the human body, *Bones, Bodies and Bellies* is just what you need. Investigations probe into how the body is put together, how the systems of the body work, and what nutrition the body needs to work efficiently. The activities are independent of each other. You can use them in any order, depending on your needs and preferences.

Bones, Bodies and Bellies should be used by "health teams" of three or four students. You may also use the activities at a learning center with individual students. The activities are designed for students in grades three through six, although they have been used with all ages of elementary students in all types of schools.

Each activity includes an introductory page that explains the concepts, lists the materials needed, and tells how to do the work, followed by one or two "labs"—pages on which students record data. The introductory page begins with a brief, concise rationale to help you focus on the main intent and to assist you in deciding the order of the activities.

The supplies that are needed for each activity are listed under the heading, "Materials." You will need to provide enough for each health team. If you present the investigations individually, place materials at a learning center, ready for the student to use. If you offer multiple investigations, or if space is limited, label and store materials and make the student responsible for gathering the supplies. The individual student should then return the materials to the proper locations after completing the activity.

Under "How to Do It," you will find suggested procedures for each investigation. This section also includes any advance preparation that may be needed. Your students may be capable of doing the preparation themselves. This is a goal you will want to strive to attain as the year advances. Special concerns and safety tips are listed in this section. Children at this age are self-conscious about their bodies. We suggest that you pair girls with girls and boys with boys on activities where there is direct body contact.

We consider "Data Collecting and Recording" a vital aspect of any lab experience. Encourage students to make and keep individual Bodylogs. Look in the section titled "Developing Bodylogs," page viii, for guidelines.

Use the Extension Activities to encourage creative problem solving and to expand the activity into a unit of study. You can assign specific extension activities or allow students to choose for themselves. Suggestions for class speakers or enrichment materials are also listed in this section.

In the Appendix, you will find blank quadrille and graph paper for recording class data. There is also a blank Table of Contents page to duplicate and include in students' Bodylogs. The Appendix also contains drawings of the hand and foot bones, which have been labeled for easy reference. Because of the increased emphasis on the whole language approach to learning, the Appendix also includes a list of relevant children's books.

Above all, when using this book, stress to students that every body is different, even though advertisers would like us to believe there is a perfect body. Create an accepting environment in your classroom so that students feel comfortable with individual differences and abilities.

Developing Bodylogs

Observations take on new meaning once they are recorded. The "Bodylogs" that your students will make as they carry out the activities in this book guide students in making and recording observations about their own bodies. Students should record only data about themselves in their Bodylogs, unless directed otherwise. The data contained in the Bodylogs can serve as a basis for comparison with other classes and grade levels. Imagine the learning that will occur as students compare the same activity later in the year (or in another year)!

The "Data Collecting and Recording" sections suggest a variety of ways to record observations. Drawings, charts, graphs, and photographs are the most common. While students may need help at first in setting up charts and graphs, it is important that they design their own as soon as possible.

Constructing graphs is a great way to integrate science and mathematics. The construction process also leads to a greater understanding of graphs and charts in other curriculum areas, such as social studies.

Data collection strategies closely resemble the way research scientists actually work. Gathering data encourages creative thought on the part of each student and helps students share information with others on their teams.

Designing the Bodylog

Although cooperative learning is the method of choice for carrying out the activities in this book, it is important that each student keep an individual Bodylog. Make class tallies and comparisons occasionally on the chalkboard or bulletin board.

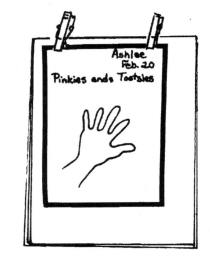

Each Bodylog is as personal as an individual's medical chart. To make this analogy more real, ask each student to bring a clipboard from home. You can also make clipboards from clothespins and several thicknesses of cardboard.

Another suggestion is to keep Bodylog papers in a manila file folder. Have each student write his or her name, last name first, on the tab. This is how clinics and hospitals keep medical files. You may consider keeping the Bodylogs in a special "medical file" or hanging them on hooks or nails if you have the room.

Following actual medical procedures will increase enthusiasm and provide motivation for the activities. Play up the health or fitness center idea. You may even want to call your students "health technicians." Encourage them to wear white coats as they do the activities. A large adult white shirt makes a good lab coat.

A complete Bodylog can also include supplemental materials, such as pamphlets available through health organizations. The student should add such materials to the Appendix.

Using the Bodylog Pages

Although we highly recommend constructing individual Bodylogs, sometimes schedules just do not allow for such creativity. If you find yourself in this situation, use the observation pages that we have included for each activity. This will standardize the Bodylogs among the teams and produce more uniform results, although it may reduce the opportunity for team creativity. Students will write their own names after "Medical Record for:" The other team members will be listed after "Practitioner(s):" For some of the activities, a student's name will appear in both places.

What to Include in the Bodylogs

A Table of Contents in the front of the Bodylog will help students locate information quickly. Simply leave the first two pages blank and fill them in as you go. Be sure to number the pages in the book as they are completed!

The activity name and date should always be included on each page of the Bodylog. Each activity has a section entitled "Data Collecting and Recording," which suggests the type of information that should be collected. You may find it helpful to discuss the method of recording data that would work best with each activity. Initially, you may even want to use a standard design. With subsequent activities, begin to allow individual planning and creative thought on the part of the "scientists." At the end of the activity, evaluate which chart or recording technique was the most effective and efficient. With long-term activities, be sure to allocate additional pages to record observations.

Students can construct simple graphs and include them right in the Bodylog. Bar graphs are easy to construct and can reveal meaningful trends. Once again, you may want to set a standard for the first one or two graphs that the class constructs.

Before you begin any data collecting, list the type of data. This will help in the design of a chart as well as remind students of the type of information they are seeking. Caution: Do not attempt to include too much in the individual Bodylogs. Combining all teams' results into a class chart or graph should be encouraged. However, a class chart is more effective when constructed as a separate activity with input from each team.

Storage of Bodylogs

You may want to consider using a special area, box, or crate for storing the individual Bodylogs. We all know that a student's desk is not the ideal location for a small, paper-bound book! At the end of the school year, each book will serve as a valuable record of the year's scientific investigations. Make your own Bodylog to provide a basis of comparison for the next year. Each year, build on the information included. In no time, you will have created a valuable resource book!

Bones

Anatomy

How We're Put Together

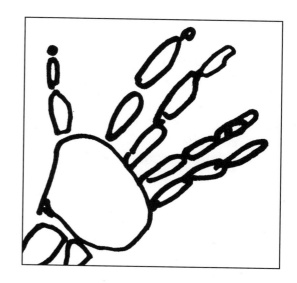

The Long and the Short of It

The framework of our bodies is made up of the bones of the body—the skeletal system. This system is vital, not only for appearance of posture, but also for blood cell production and muscle movement. This activity offers an opportunity to study the skeletal system from a different perspective. By measuring and comparing individual bones, students begin to see why certain bones are called long and others short.

Materials

    String
    Measuring sticks or tapes (in yards or meters)
    Pencils
    Bodylog or Paper

How to Do It

We recommend you divide teams into pairs of the same gender because of the direct physical contact required in this activity. If a posterboard skeleton is available, use it as your guide. If none is available, use a picture of a skeleton from a current science or health book. Students should refer to the picture as they measure their own bodies. Starting with the appendages (arms and legs), measure each bone from tip to tip. For example, lift the upper arm to find the top tip of the humerus (upper arm). Then move the elbow to define the lower tip of the bone. Measure each bone of the appendages the same way. When measuring the bones of the hands and feet, students will have to probe for the ends of the metacarpals (hand bones) and metatarsals (foot bones). Use the string to determine length. Then hold the string against the measuring stick for actual size.

Data Collecting and Recording

Measure as many long and short bones as possible. Remember, there are two bones in the lower leg—the fibula, the bone on the outside (the bottom tip is the outside ankle), and the tibia, the bone on the inside (the bottom tip is the inside ankle). Record all values in the Bodylog.

Compare all the numbers and identify the long bones based on actual data. Find the longest bone in the body. Compare the sizes of bones. Find this bone on each member of the class. If students understand percentages, determine the longest bone as a percent of the whole body height.

Extension Activities

- Make skeleton mobiles using string lengths to represent actual bone lengths. Attach the strings to a cardboard torso.
- Compare bone lengths with other classes and grade levels.
- Devise a system for measuring the irregular bones (pelvis, vertebrae, wrist, and foot bones) and flat bones (skull and shoulder blades).
- Contact a hospital or doctor and ask for old X-rays (even if only on loan). Hang them against the windows where all can see. Find the bones you see in the X-rays on the model skeleton and on a human body.
- Attempt to draw the bones using the correct measurements. Construct individual life-sized bones.
- Ask a butcher to save cow or pig bones for examination and comparison.
- Invite a chiropractor to your room to speak on her occupation.
- "Pinkies and Tootsies" on page 14 is a related activity that you will want to try.

Medical Record for: _____

Practitioner(s): _____ Date: _____

The Long and Short of It

Practitioner note: Find and record the details for as many bones as possible.

BONE NAME and/or LOCATION	LENGTH	CATEGORY Long, Short, Flat, or Irregular	OTHER DATA

Straight as a Board

The vertebral column (backbone) helps us stand up straight and carry loads. The backbone also supports the spinal cord, which carries nerve transmissions from the brain to the rest of the body. Awareness of the backbone's structure and function may direct students to care for their vertebral columns early, to prevent damage later in life.

How would we be different if the backbone was one bone, like the femur in the upper leg? This activity graphically shows how a backbone composed of several smaller bones gives us the ability to bend.

Materials

Straws (2)
Yarn (2 pieces, approximately 1 meter each)
Scissors
Protractor (optional)
Bodylog or paper
Pencil

How to Do It

Use a straw to represent the vertebral column and a piece of yarn to represent the spinal cord. Thread the yarn through the straw and tie the ends together. Cut a second straw into 10 equal pieces. Thread another piece of yarn through all of the pieces. Tie the ends together.

Data Collecting and Recording

Compare the flexibility of the two straw backbones. Lay the backbones side by side. Can both backbones be made straight? Which backbone can be made to curve without bending the straw? Make sure the "vertebrae" are next to each other (touching) in the backbone made from 10 straw pieces. What happens to the spinal cord running through the complete straw if you bend the straw?

In the Bodylog, trace the curve of the straw backbones. If your students know how to use a protractor, have them determine the degree of the curve.

Extension Activities

- Cut the straw pieces to scale of the vertebrae in an actual vertebral column. Where is the backbone the most flexible?

- "Stick Your Neck Out!," page 8, and "The Flex Test," page 26, make excellent extension activities.

- Ask your local butcher to save poultry and cattle vertebrae for you. Can you reassemble the backbones?

- Ask a chiropractor for information on the backbone. He may have some brochures or models that he would let you borrow.

- Encourage good posture in the classroom. Have students do a "posture check" several times during the day.

From *Bones, Bodies and Bellies*, published by GoodYearBooks. Copyright © 1994 Diane A. Vaszily and Peggy K. Perdue.

Straight as a Board

Practitioner note: Please draw patients' vertebral columns below.

"Patient A's" Vertebral Column (with one vertebrae)	"Patient B's" Vertebral Column (with 10 vertebrae)

On the back of this form, trace how far Patient A can bend with one solid vertebra. Do the same for Patient B with 10 vertebrae. (Note: Make sure each vertebra is touching the one beside it.)

In your opinion, why is it important that our backbones be made of several vertebrae?

_____

_____

Stick Your Neck Out!

The neck is a sensitive area of the anatomy. It is the main highway for messages between the brain and the rest of the body. Damage to the neck can cause paralysis or even death. The neck is at the top of the vertebral column, which provides protection to the spinal cord.

When you look at a giraffe, it's hard to miss the great length of its neck. In fact, the neck of a giraffe can be almost one-third of its length! It's hard to believe, but giraffes and humans both have seven neck bones. In this activity, students will examine their necks and compare them to their vertebral columns.

Materials

Washable marker
Model or picture of vertebral column
Full-length mirror (optional)
Hand-held mirror (optional)
Calculator
Bodylog or paper
Pencils

How to Do It

We recommend that you divide teams into pairs of the same gender because of the direct physical contact required in this activity. Boys should work with boys, and girls should work with girls.

Ask students to wear swimming suits under their school clothes on the day you plan to do this activity. Have each student bend over as if to touch his or her toes. Using the washable marker, the student's partner should make a dot on the part of each vertebra that protrudes near the surface of the skin. This part of the vertebra is called the process. Use caution in the neck area. Because the processes here may be too small to locate, use a skeleton model or a picture. The neck consists of seven cervical vertebrae.

After marking each process, have students stand erect and count the marks. Attempt to designate the four areas of the vertebral column. Starting at the top, there are seven cervical vertebrae, twelve thoracic vertebrae, five lumbar, and five sacral vertebrae. The sacral vertebrae are usually fused; only the top one will be visible.

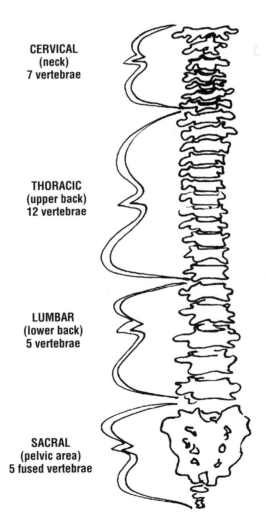

**CERVICAL
(neck)
7 vertebrae**

**THORACIC
(upper back)
12 vertebrae**

**LUMBAR
(lower back)
5 vertebrae**

**SACRAL
(pelvic area)
5 fused vertebrae**

From *Bones, Bodies and Bellies*, published by GoodYearBooks. Copyright © 1994 Diane A. Vaszily and Peggy K. Perdue.

Data Collecting and Recording

Measure the entire length of the vertebral column. Record the length in the Bodylog. Compare the neck length to the length of the entire vertebral column. Find the percentage. If your students are unable to do the calculations by hand, they may use calculators.

Use this formula:

(Neck Length/Overall Length of vertebral column) x 100

Example:

Neck length = 3 inches	Overall length = 36 inches
(3/36) x 100 = 8.33%	
The neck is approximately 8% of the vertebral column	

You can analyze each section of vertebrae and calculate its percentage of the whole spinal column. Use the same formula. Substitute the length of the area being measured for "neck length" in the formula. Record all findings in the Bodylog.

Extension Activities

■ Is the ratio of neck to vertebral column the same in males and females? Compare the percentages in your class.

■ Does the neck percentage increase with age? Compare younger children for neck length percentage to parents and, if possible, grandparents.

■ Make a model of a vertebral column using the correct number of Life Savers®, thread spools, or round discs. Place felt pads between each "disc" to simulate the cartilaginous discs. If you use Life Savers®, use a different color to represent each area of the vertebral column.

Medical Record for: _____

Practitioner(s): _____   Date: _____

Stick Your Neck Out

Practitioner note: Draw the shape of the patient's vertebral column from the dots on his or her back. Is the vertebral column straight?

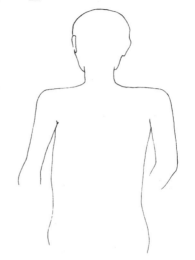

CERVICAL	Number of vertebrae in neck	
	Length of cervical area	
	Percentage of total length	
THORACIC	Number of vertebrae in upper back	
	Length of thoracic area	
	Percentage of total length	
LUMBAR	Number of vertebrae in lower back	
	Length of lumbar area	
	Percentage of total length	
SACRAL	Number of vertebrae in pelvic area	
	Length of sacral area	
	Percentage of total length	

From *Bones, Bodies and Bellies*, published by GoodYearBooks. Copyright © 1994 Diane A. Vaszily and Peggy K. Perdue.

From Ear to Ear

Ears! We hear with them, adorn them with jewelry, and use them to hold on glasses. Does heredity play a part in ear placement? When working with genetics, students often examine eye and hair color. Why not examine the unusual? In this activity, students will examine the placement of the ears in relationship to other parts of the face and head and attempt to relate ear placement to heredity.

Materials

Measuring tape or yarn and a measuring stick
Goggles (optional)
Overhead or slide projector
Dark construction paper (11" x 18")
Tape
Paper for ear
Scissors
Mirror
Bodylogs
Pencil
Sweat band

How to Do It

Because students will be working near the eyes, we advise that they wear safety goggles for protection.

Before beginning, place a sweat band around the center of the forehead on each child to be measured. Use the same type of sweat band so the sizes are uniform. For the first measurement, place one end of the yarn at the center point of the left ear and extend the yarn up the side to the top of the sweat band. Record the measurement. Repeat on the right side. Measure the length of the yarn used. Use that measurement to place the ear.

Next, measure from the center of one ear to the center of the bridge of the nose (do not round the front of the face). Measure the length of yarn used. Repeat, using the other ear. Use this measure to place the ear.

From *Bones, Bodies and Bellies*, published by GoodYearBooks. Copyright © 1994 Diane A. Vaszily and Peggy K. Perdue.

Data Collecting and Recording

Use an overhead or filmstrip projector to make silhouettes of each child. The student should sit sideways between the overhead and a wall. To get a more accurate head size, the student should be close to the wall. Adjust the projector until the image projected onto the wall is sharp. Attach a dark sheet of construction paper to the wall. Trace the shadow made by the student's head. Cut out the silhouette. Using the measurements gathered, place a paper cut-out ear at the correct location. If a smaller size is desired to place in the Bodylog, use a copier to reduce the silhouette until it can fit onto the Bodylog page. An alternative method is to draw the head to scale on quadrille paper.

Compare measurements among classmates. How similar is ear placement?

Make measurements on siblings, parents, and other relatives to determine if heredity is a factor.

Extension Activities

■ Compare numbers compiled by girls versus boys. Is there any trend that can be identified?

■ How the ear is attached to the head is also an inherited trait. Have students look at ear lobes. Are they attached (a recessive trait) or free (a dominant trait)? Compare with classmates and family members.

■ Another inherited trait is a point on the pinna (the outside part) of the ear. An ear point present on the pinna is a dominate trait. No ear point on the pinna is recessive. Have students examine classmates' ears and those of family members. Is there a correlation?

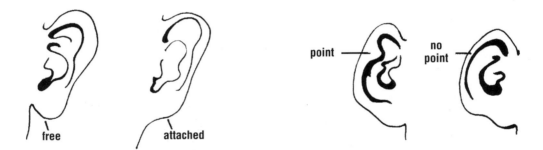

■ Contact an ear specialist for models of ears. She may be willing to spend time in your classroom sharing models and photographs and answering questions.

From *Bones, Bodies and Bellies*, published by GoodYearBooks. Copyright © 1994 Diane A. Vaszily and Peggy K. Perdue.

Medical Record for: _____

Practitioner(s): _____ Date: _____

From Ear to Ear

Practitioner note: Draw or attach patient's profile below.

Location	Measurement
Ear to Sweatband (left/right)	
Bridge of Nose to Left Ear	
Bridge of Nose to Right Ear	

Draw the shape of the patient's ear.

Pinkies and Tootsies

Over half of the bones in our bodies are found in our hands and feet! Since we were babies, we have been counting fingers, sending piggies to market, and placing rings on pinkies. Even with this familiarity, the anatomy of our hands and feet is often a mystery covered by skin. This activity will end the mystery as students count and measure the bones that make up their feet and hands.

Materials

Measuring tape or string and ruler
Plain paper to trace hand and foot (3 pieces)
Pictures of hand skeleton and foot skeleton for reference (See pages 83 and 84 in the Appendix.)
Bodylog or paper
Pencil

How to Do It

Trace a hand on a sheet of paper and a foot on another. The tracing of the foot should include a side view as well as a top view (use another piece of paper if necessary). Next, measure the bones in the phalanges (fingers and toes) from end to end. A joint, or where the phalanx bends, indicates the end of the bone. Draw the bone in its proper location on the tracing. Attempt to find each metacarpal (hand bone) and measure it. Draw the carpal bones of the wrist. Do the same with the foot. The metatarsals are the foot bones and the tarsals are in the ankle.

Data Collecting

The bone length of each digit and toe should be recorded in the Bodylog. This could be done right on the tracings or on a chart that is included with the tracings. A dramatic representation is to make the hand and foot tracing on black paper and cut the bones from white paper. Glue the white paper onto the black, one bone at a time.

Extension Activities

■ Plan this activity for late October and you'll have your Halloween decorations!

■ Compare the digit length from child to child. Compare body height to finger length. Is there a relationship?

■ Ask a radiologist for X-rays of hands and feet. Measure the bones and compare.

■ Contact a podiatrist. He may have models, posters, or brochures that he would like to share with your class.

Medical Record for: _____

Practitioner(s): _____   Date: _____

Pinkies and Tootsies

Practitioner note: When measuring the phalanges (bones of the fingers and toes), start with the one closest to the nail and work toward the palm. Remember, the thumb, big toe, and little toe only have two bones each!

LEFT HAND			
Little Finger			
Ring Finger			
Middle Finger			
Pointer Finger			
Thumb			

Total Length of Hand (from fingertip to wrist) _____

RIGHT HAND			
Little Finger			
Ring Finger			
Middle Finger			
Pointer Finger			
Thumb			

Total Length of Hand (from fingertip to wrist) _____

LEFT FOOT			
Big Toe			
Second Toe			
Third Toe			
Fourth Toe			
Little Toe			

Total Length of Foot (from end of toe to ankle) _____

RIGHT FOOT			
Big Toe			
Second Toe			
Third Toe			
Fourth Toe			
Little Toe			

Total Length of Foot (from end of toe to ankle) _____

Is one hand larger than the other? Which one? _____

Is one foot larger than the other? Which one? _____

If there is a difference, is the larger bone located on the same side for both the hand and foot? Compare your findings with colleagues.

From *Bones, Bodies and Bellies*, published by GoodYearBooks. Copyright © 1994 Diane A. Vaszily and Peggy K. Perdue.

Arch Rivals

Our feet carry all of our weight wherever we want to go. For feet to work properly and feel good, shoes must fit correctly. One measurement that is made to determine shoe size is the position of the arch. In this activity, students will be making footprints to examine the arches in their feet. Students will definitely remember the day they painted their feet in class!

Materials

Tempera or other water-based paint
Plastic
Bulletin board or freezer paper
Water
Towels
Ruler
Bodylog or paper
Quadrille paper (optional—see page 80 in the Appendix)
Scissors (optional)
Pencil

How to Do It

Note: Some children may not have an arch. This is not a defect; some arches are late to form. Before beginning this activity, make sure that water and towels are available for clean-up.

For each student, place a piece of plastic on the floor. Put a piece of bulletin board or freezer paper on top. Pour a small amount of paint onto the paper. Have students step into the paint with one bare foot. Students should then step onto the white paper. Clean the painted foot and repeat the process with the other foot. Have students label the footprints with their name, date, and which foot the print represents. Allow the prints to dry.

If you choose not to use paint, you can still do this activity. Have each child bring a large sponge and a large plastic bag from home. Wet the sponge and place it on the plastic bag on the floor. Have students carefully step barefooted onto the sponge, then onto the paper. Trace around the footprint with chalk.

Data Collecting and Recording

Have students measure and record the length and width of their prints. To measure the arch, draw a straight line from the ball area of the foot to the heel. The line should touch the outermost points of the print. Measure the length and width of the arch. Repeat for the other print.

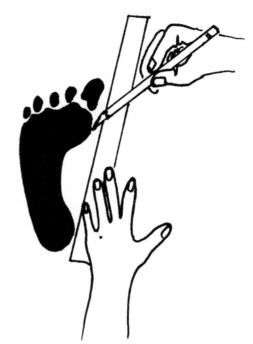

For a more accurate measurement, cut out the print and place it on a piece of quadrille paper. Trace around the print. Once again, draw a straight line from the ball area of the foot to the heel. Determine the area by counting the squares between the drawn line and the tracing of the print. Count all whole squares and those that have more than half of their area within the lines. Older students may be able to calculate the percentage the arch is of the entire footprint.

Extension Activities

- Ask to borrow a foot sizer from a shoe store. Have students practice measuring their feet. Are both feet the same?
- Invite a podiatrist into the class to share information on proper foot care.
- Discuss the importance of shoes that fit properly.
- Compare the length and width of the arch to that of the entire foot. Is there any correlation?
- Analyze shoes with arches. What size are the arches? Which types of shoes contain arches and which do not? Which rest your feet more—shoes with or without arches?

From *Bones, Bodies and Bellies*, published by GoodYearBooks. Copyright © 1994 Diane A. Vaszily and Peggy K. Perdue.

Lab

Medical Record for: _____

Practitioner(s): _____ Date: _____

Arch Rivals

FOOT PRINT

Practitioner note: Put patient's footprint here or use page 84, "Foot Bones." Be sure to label it "Left Foot" or "Right Foot."

     To measure the arch, draw a straight line from the ball area of the foot to the heel. The line should touch the outermost points of the print.

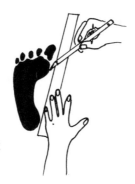

LEFT FOOT	
AREA MEASURED	**MEASUREMENT**
Length of Foot	
Width of Foot	
Length of Arch	
Width of Arch	

RIGHT FOOT	
AREA MEASURED	**MEASUREMENT**
Length of Foot	
Width of Foot	
Length of Arch	
Width of Arch	

Seeing Eye to Eye

Eyes are windows to the world, indicators of good health, expressions of mood, and signs of beauty. The tasks they perform are varied. Students will become involved in analyzing and comparing physical characteristics of eyes as well as their functions.

Materials

Yarn and ruler or a measuring tape
Index card 3" x 5"
Mirror
Crayons or colored pencils
Bodylog or paper
Pencil

How to Do It

Eye Placement

Caution: It is advisable to wear a set of safety goggles while making measurements near the eye. Measure the distance from the outside edge of each eye to the center of the bridge of the nose. Look in a mirror and determine eye shape.

Note: Eye shape is often associated with race. Use caution when discussing eye placement with children.

Color

The iris is the colored portion of the eye. Try to reproduce the color (or colors) of the iris by using crayons or pastels. You may need to blend colors to achieve a perfect match.

Peripheral Vision

Hold the index card in front of the eyes. Move the card around to the side until you can no longer see it. During this activity, the eyes must focus straight ahead and not look to the side.

Focus Length

Hold a card with a small line of type in front of the eyes. Bring the card close to the eyes. The type should become blurry. Slowly move the card away from the eyes until the line of type is clear. Continue moving the card farther until the type becomes blurry again. The Focus Length is the range where the type is clear.

From *Bones, Bodies and Bellies*, published by GoodYearBooks. Copyright © 1994 Diane A. Vaszily and Peggy K. Perdue.

Data Collecting and Recording

Draw the eye placement in the Bodylog. Be sure to make careful measurements. Would the eyes be classified as close together or far apart? Attempt to draw the eye shape in your Bodylog.

Reproduce eye color in the Bodylog. Look for special markings. Is there a ring around the pupil (the dark circle in the eye) that is a different color? Is the outside edge of the iris the same color or is it darker? Is the iris one color, or does it have shading?

For peripheral vision, determine what part of a 360° circle each student can see. Mark it in the Bodylog. (This is a good time to introduce a protractor and degrees of a circle.)

Measure the focal range with a measuring stick. Record the closest and the farthest distance from the eye that the type is clear.

Extension Activities

■ How does color affect peripheral vision? Repeat the experiment above, using different colors of index cards or construction paper. Make sure that the card size is consistent.

■ Compare the results of this activity with others in the class. How do boys compare with girls?

■ Does age make a difference in the test results? Have students make observations on family members. Bring the results to class. Make a graph including everyone's data.

■ Invite an optometrist or ophthalmologist into your room. Many have slides on the eye.

Medical Record for: _____

Practitioner(s): _____ Date: _____

Seeing Eye to Eye

Patient Eye Chart

Eye Placement

Practitioner note: Where are the patient's eyes in relation to the nose? Measure from the center of the bridge of the nose to the closest corner of the left eye. Measure from the center of the bridge of the nose to the far corner of the left eye. Repeat for the right eye. Draw patient's eyes here.

Eye Color

Practitioner note: Look at patient's eyes. Look for special markings. Is there a ring around the pupil (the dark circle in the eye) that is a different color? Is the outside edge of the iris the same color? Is the iris one color, or does it have shading? Record your findings below.

Peripheral Vision

Practitioner note: Hold the index card in front of the eyes, about an arm's length away. Move the card around to the left side until the patient can no longer see it. Repeat, but move the card to the right side. Remember that the eyes must focus straight ahead and not look to the side.

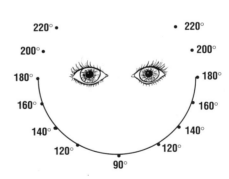

Focus Length

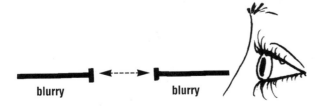

Practitioner note: Hold a card with a small line of type in front of the patient's eyes. The card should be close to the eyes and the type blurry. Slowly move the card away from the eyes until the line of type is clear to the patient. Measure the distance. Continue moving the card farther until the type becomes blurry again. Measure the distance. The Focus Length is the range where the type is clear. Record your findings.

From *Bones, Bodies and Bellies*, published by GoodYearBooks. Copyright © 1994 Diane A. Vaszily and Peggy K. Perdue.

22

Sockets and Hinges

How do we move? Our 206 bones give us movement by their pivoting mechanisms. Joints provide ease of movement. They can "stiffen up" due to muscle strain. Students will be made more aware of joints and their role in mobility by attempting to locate and classify the joints in their bodies.

Materials

Hinge (a doorway provides a good look at hinge action)
Ball and socket joint (the leg bone and hip of a chicken after cooking and deboning)
Bodylog or paper
Pencil

How to Do It

There are six types of joints in the human body: ball and socket, hinge, slightly moveable, immovable, gliding, and pivot. Immovable joints do not move. Each of the other types allows a different type of movement. In this activity, students will identify ball and socket joints and hinge joints.

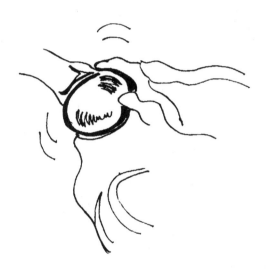

Start with a demonstration on the type of movement the two joints allow. Have students examine how the chicken bones come together (ball and socket joint). Ask what type of movement the joint would allow. Students should notice that a wide range of movement is allowed with this type of joint.

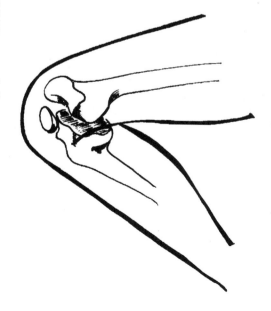

Now have students examine the hinge. What type of movement is allowed? A hinge joint allows movement in only one direction.

Next have students examine their own bodies. Where is movement allowed? Start with the fingers, move to the wrists and up the arms. Do the same with the toes, ankles, and legs. What type of movement is allowed at each joint?

Data Collecting and Recording

Students should record the location of each Ball and Socket joint and each Hinge joint in their Bodylog. How many of each type do they find?

Extension Activities

■ Have students investigate what the other types of joints are called in the body. Can they find examples of each? (immovable joint—skull; slightly moveable—vertebrae; pivot—atlas and axis bones in neck; gliding—wrist)

■ We often oil joints in mechanical devices to keep them working properly. Investigate what lubricates the joints in our bodies (synovial fluid).

■ Ask a butcher to save cattle or other animal joints that she might have. Do joints vary from animal to animal?

■ Ask a radiologist or a veterinarian to save X-rays for you. Display the X-rays around the room.

■ There are more than 200 joints in your body. Try not using four. Pretend that there are no joints at your elbows and knees. Legs and arms must be kept straight. Discuss how you feel after 10 minutes.

From *Bones, Bodies and Bellies*, published by GoodYearBooks. Copyright © 1994 Diane A. Vaszily and Peggy K. Perdue.

Lab	Medical Record for: _____
	Practitioner(s): _____ Date: _____

Sockets and Hinges

Practitioner note: Find where the hinge and the ball and socket joints are hidden in the body. Start with the fingers, move to the wrists and up the arms. Do the same with the toes, ankles, and legs. Write the location of the hinge joints and the ball and socket joints that you find.

Joint Number	Location of Hinge Joint

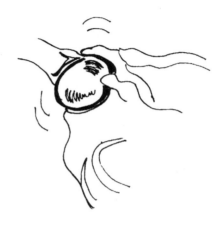

Joint Number	Location of Ball and Socket Joint

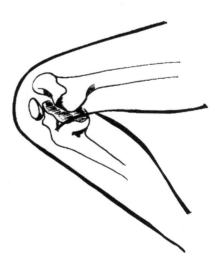

The Flex Test

Before participating in any sport, a "warm-up" is necessary. This stretches muscles and reduces the chances of injury. Some people seem to be born flexible. Others have little flexibility. Most people are somewhere in the middle. Flexibility is important, and humans can become more limber. In this activity, students will measure their flexibility and then work to increase it.

Materials

Measuring tape or string and yardstick
Mat
Bodylog or paper
Pencil

How to Do It

Tuck loose shirts into pants. Remind girls to wear shorts or pants on the day that measurements will be made.

Students will do a series of four activities to determine flexibility. Students should work in pairs; one student to do the activity, the second student to take and record the measurement. Students should then switch responsibilities.

For the first activity, have students sit on the floor with their legs straight and as far apart as possible. Students should slowly lower their chests toward the floor. Backs should be kept straight.

Have students stand with feet together and knees straight. Students should slowly bend from the waist and try to touch their toes with their fingertips.

Students should stand, using the back of a chair for support and balance. Raise the left leg as high to the side as possible. Repeat using the right leg.

The next activity should be done with a mat. Have students lay with their backs on the mat, knees bent, feet flat on mat. Put palms of hands on mat near ears. Fingers should be close to the shoulders. Students should push gently from their feet and hands to raise their bodies into a bridge.

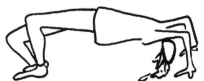

From Bones, Bodies and Bellies, published by GoodYearBooks. Copyright © 1994 Diane A. Vaszily and Peggy K. Perdue.

Data Collecting and Recording

On the first test, measure from the shoulders to the floor. Measure how close the hands are to the floor on the toe touch test. If students can touch the floor with their fingertips, see if they can place their hands flat on the floor. On the leg lift, measure the distance between the heel and the floor. Be sure to measure both legs as the results could be different. For the bridge test, measure the distance between the waist and the floor. All measurements should be recorded in the Bodylog.

Invite the physical education teacher or a coach to show the students appropriate stretching exercises. Encourage students to do the exercises every day. Take new measurements every other week for several weeks. Use a line graph to record the results. Is flexibility increasing?

Extension Activities

- Compare statistics. Which sex appears more flexible?
- Does age influence flexibility? Get the whole family involved in the activity. Can everyone improve their flexibility?
- Videotape warm-up exercises for various sports. Your high school may already have the videos and all you will need to do is request copies. There are also warm-ups on most exercise tapes. Show the videos. Identify the muscles being stretched.
- Try the flex test at various times during the day. When is flexibility the greatest? The least?
- Invite a doctor specializing in sports medicine to be a guest in the classroom. What injuries are most prevalent?

Medical Record for: _____

Practitioner(s): _____   Date: _____

The Flex Test

Patient Flexibility Record

Flex Test #1: Chest to floor

Practitioner note: Have the patient sit on the floor with legs straight and as far apart as possible. The patient should slowly lower chest toward the floor, keeping the back straight. Measure the distance from the shoulders to the floor.

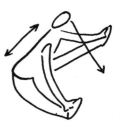

Flex Test #2: Toe Touch

Practitioner note: Have the patient stand with feet together and knees straight. Then have the patient slowly bend from the waist and try to touch the toes with the fingertips. Measure how close the hands are to the floor. Can the patient place his or her hands flat on the floor?

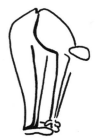

Flex Test #3: Leg Lift

Practitioner note: Have the patient stand, using the back of a chair for support and balance. Then have the patient raise the left leg as high to the side as possible. Repeat, using the right leg. Measure the distance between the heel and the floor. Be sure to measure both legs as the results could be different.

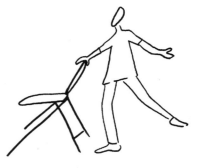

Flex Test #4: Bridge

Practitioner note: Have the patient use a mat and lie with his or her back on the mat, with knees bent and feet flat on the mat. Ask the patient to put the palms of the hands on the mat near the ears, with the fingers close to the shoulders. The patient should push up gently from the feet and hands to raise the body into a bridge. Measure the distance between the waist and the floor.

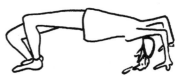

Record results on chart.

Test	Distance From Floor
Chest to Floor	
Toe Touch	
Leg Lift	
Bridge	

From *Bones, Bodies and Bellies*, published by GoodYearBooks. Copyright © 1994 Diane A. Vaszily and Peggy K. Perdue.

Bodies

Physiology

How We Work

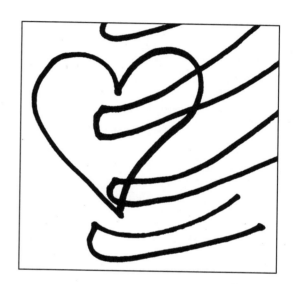

Revving Up the Engine

A healthy heart is capable of long periods of strenuous exercise without speeding up excessively. It should return to its normal pulse rate in five minutes. Keeping a heart healthy depends as much on exercise as it does on diet. This activity will help students use pulse rate to determine their level of fitness.

Materials

Stopwatch or watch with second hand for each team
Exercise course (stairs, treadmill, track, or a spacious room for exercising)

How to Do It

Caution students to progress slowly when beginning an exercise program. Students should choose an exercise that corresponds with their ability.

It is absolutely essential that each student know how to take a pulse—either at the wrist, neck, or temple. Have them practice for several minutes before doing this activity. Quiet, accurate counting is essential. Students can count for 60 seconds, although many will lose count over this period of time. Another way is to count the pulse rate for 6 seconds and then multiply by 10.

Have each student take their pulse rate at a quiet, restful time of the day (not after returning from gym, lunch, or recess!). Take pulse several times during the day so an average can be attained.

Set up an exercise course that can be used for testing. Decide on how long the students will exercise. Three to five minutes is sufficient for raising heart rate.

Data Collecting and Recording

The first pulse taken is the resting heart rate. Record it in the Bodylog at the 0 line. After exercise, a healthy heart should return to the at-rest rate as quickly as possible. The time it takes the heart to return to the at-rest rate is known as the recovery rate.

Immediately after the exercise time has elapsed, have each student take his or her pulse for 6 seconds. Approximately 55 seconds later, take the pulse again. Continue to take the pulse for 6 seconds at 55-second intervals until the heart rate returns to normal. You may wish to have students refrain from doing computation of beats per minute until they have completed taking all of the pulse readings.

It may take days or weeks of repeating this procedure to reduce the recovery rate, but an exercise schedule should be maintained to do just that. Record all the pulse readings in the Bodylog over several weeks.

Extension Activities

- Compare pulse rates and recovery rates for different age levels.
- Try this activity with athletes and non-athletes. How do the results compare?
- Plan an exercise program and use it for one month. Monitor pulse rates.

From *Bones, Bodies and Bellies*, published by GoodYearBooks. Copyright © 1994 Diane A. Vaszily and Peggy K. Perdue.

Medical Record for: _____

Practitioner(s): _____ Date: _____

Revving Up the Engine

Vital Signs Record

Practitioner note: Take patient's pulse at rest. Have patient exercise 3 to 5 minutes. Take pulse every minute until pulse is back to resting rate. Record pulse rates below.

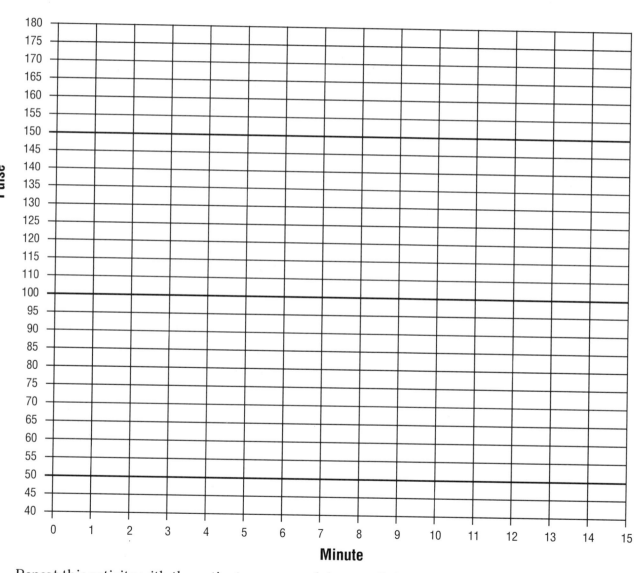

Repeat this activity with the patient over several days until the pulse rate is back to the at-rest rate within 5 minutes. Use a different color line for each day. Include a key.

Cold Noses

Body temperature is an indicator of health or illness. A narrow range exists within which a warm-blooded body will function effectively. The body employs mechanisms for maintaining these temperatures. The hypothalamus gland regulates temperatures in the human body. Students will gather temperatures from various areas of the body and establish that area's "norm."

Materials

Tape thermometer or oral thermometer and probe covers for each team
Bodylog
Pencil

How to Do It

Caution: If you are using an oral thermometer, it is crucial that you use disposable probe covers. Students should handle only their own probe covers.

Students should be able to read a thermometer before doing this activity. Take a few minutes to review this skill if necessary.

Place students in teams of the same gender. Boys should be with boys and girls should be with girls.

Assign a variety of spots at which to take temperatures—inside the mouth (if using an oral thermometer), forehead (if using a tape thermometer), under the armpit, inside a closed fist, on the tip of the nose, against the stomach or abdominal area, behind the knee, and between the toes.

Data Collecting and Recording

Have each student record the temperature at all the locations listed on the chart. On the board, or on a large piece of bulletin-board paper, make a class chart. Each student should be responsible for recording his/her data on the chart.

Is there a difference in temperature from mid-body to extremities? Determine the lowest temperature location on the body.

Extension Activities

■   Take temperature readings at the same body locations when the temperatures are cooler (outdoors during the winter months or indoors in an air-conditioned room).

■   Take temperature at rest and after exercise (or an active gym or recess period). Is there any variation in the body temperature?

■   Take temperatures at different times of the day (immediately after rising, at noon, and right before bed).

From *Bones, Bodies and Bellies*, published by GoodYearBooks. Copyright © 1994 Diane A. Vaszily and Peggy K. Perdue.

Cold Noses

Vital Signs Record

Practitioner note: Identify the exact locations of temperature readings on the figure below. Then fill out the chart.

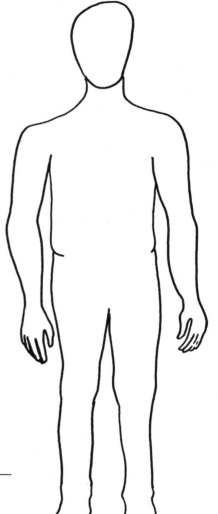

LOCATION	TEMPERATURE	TYPE OF THERMOMETER
Inside Mouth		Oral Thermometer
Forehead		Tape Thermometer
Under Arm		
Closed Fist		
Tip of Nose		
Waist Area		
Behind Knee		
Toes		

What area of the patient's body is the coldest? _____

What area of the patient's body is the warmest? _____

Don't Hold Your Breath

Proper breathing is a requirement for good air exchange, but many people are unaware of the need for total air exchange (exhaling all of the carbon dioxide in the body and replacing it with oxygen). Students will determine their own lung capacity, called vital capacity, by exhaling as much air as possible from the lungs. The exhaled air will displace an equal amount of water, making this measurement possible.

Materials

Basin large enough to hold 2 gallons of water (1 per team)

One-gallon milk jug for each team, marked on one side at one-inch intervals. Start numbering at the neck and work toward the bottom of the jug.

A three-foot length of tubing (aquarium tubing) for each student. An alternate method is to have each student place a clean straw inside the same tube. It must be airtight for the experiment to work.

An accurate measuring device, such as a measuring cup, a beaker, or a graduated cylinder

Water

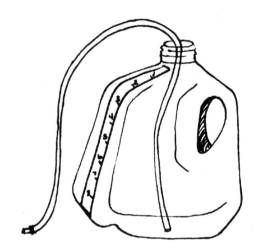

How to Do It

Fill the jug to the brim with water. Put on the cap or hold your hand over the top of the opening. Immerse the jug upside down in a basin of water filled to a depth of two inches.

Remove the cap of the inverted vital capacity bottle and place one end of the tube into the jug. Place the straw in the other end of the tube. The straw goes into the student's mouth.

Have the student take a deep breath. Exhale into the straw/tube slowly until no more air can be forced out of the student's lungs. Then exhale again without taking a breath! The air going into the jug will displace a like amount of water. Have each student do three trials.

From *Bones, Bodies and Bellies*, published by GoodYearBooks. Copyright © 1994 Diane A. Vaszily and Peggy K. Perdue.

Data Collecting and Recording

Determine how much water the filled jug will hold. It should be a gallon or 3,840 cc. After exhaling, determine how much is left in the jug and calculate the amount of water that was displaced. The formula is:

(Water in full jug) - (Water left in jug) = Water Displaced

Vital capacity is usually measured in cubic centimeters (cc). One ounce of water equals 30 ml or 30 cubic centimeters. Record the three trials in the body log. You may wish to have students determine their average vital capacity ([Trial #1 + Trial #2 + Trial #3]/3). Make a class chart and graph showing vital capacities.

Extension Activities

■ Compare vital capacities to chest circumference. Is there a relationship?

■ Compare vital capacities to age. Choose five-year age differences. You may need to have a second jug ready for those who can empty the first and still have more residual air.

■ Ask a hospital if they could provide a vital capacity apparatus for the class to observe.

Don't Hold Your Breath

Vital Signs Record

Practitioner note: Fill jug with water and cap. Turn the jug upside-down and lower into a basin of water. Remove the cap. Place one end of the tube into the jug. Place a straw in the other end of the tube. Have the patient take a deep breath and exhale into the straw slowly until no more air can be forced out the lungs. The water displaced from the jug will equal the patient's vital capacity. Record vital capacity on the chart. Remember to add the unit of measure (cc).

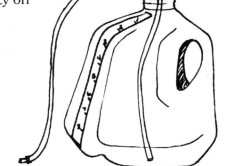

TRIAL NUMBER	VITAL CAPACITY
1	
2	
3	

Practitioner note: You may wish to confer with your colleagues on their patients and compare their results. Record your findings on the chart below.

PATIENT	VITAL CAPACITY TRIAL #1	VITAL CAPACITY TRIAL #2	VITAL CAPACITY TRIAL #3

From *Bones, Bodies and Bellies*, published by GoodYearBooks. Copyright © 1994 Diane A. Vaszily and Peggy K. Perdue.

Prickle Puzzles

We feel pain, pressure, and temperature because of specific nerve receptors located within our skin. Nerve endings fan out to cover most of the surface area of the body. The endings are more dense in areas of greater need. This activity will allow students to predict which areas of the skin's surface are more sensitive (and therefore have more nerve endings).

Materials

Blindfold
Pointed toothpicks (2 per student)
Metric ruler
Scrap paper
Rubber band or tape
Body chart from Bodylog
Pencil

How to Do It

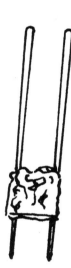

Caution students to press the toothpicks gently onto the skin. Also, pair students into teams of the same gender to prevent excess silliness.

Use wadded paper to space the toothpicks 5 mm apart. Tape or rubber band the toothpicks together. Work in teams of two; one student is the subject and one is the tester. Blindfold the subject before beginning. The tester then touches areas of the subject's skin with one or two toothpick points. The subject indicates when he or she feels the pressure of the touch and whether it is with one or two points. The tester could say, "Do you feel pressure?" "One or two points?" The tester should test with two points and one point in a random fashion.

Data Collecting and Recording

If nerve endings are spaced far apart, the subject will feel only one point, even though the tester is using both points against the skin.

Indicate at each point tested on the Bodylog diagram whether the subject felt one point (marked with the numeral 1) or two points (marked with the numeral 2). If no feeling occurred, use an X. If the subject correctly identified the number of points, draw a circle around the number.

From *Bones, Bodies and Bellies*, published by GoodYearBooks. Copyright © 1994 Diane A. Vaszily and Peggy K. Perdue.

Extension Activities

■ Vary the distance the toothpicks are held apart to 1 cm. Test the same areas again. Is there a difference in the results?

■ Test subjects of different ages.

■ Test subjects who work outside in the sun. Is there a difference between them and those who work inside?

■ Test for temperature sensitivity on the skin. Straighten one end of a metal paper clip. Hold the end in ice water for 10 seconds. Touch the cold end to one of the areas that was tested in the above activity. Repeat for each location. Which areas are sensitive to cold? Repeat using hot water to warm the end of the metal paper clip. Compare the results.

Medical Record for: _____

Practitioner(s): _____ Date: _____

Prickle Puzzles

Sensitivity Record Form

Practitioner note: Label each spot that you test on your patient. If patient feels one point, write the numeral 1 on the spot. If patient feels two points, write the numeral 2. If patient feels no points, mark the spot with an X. If the response is correct, draw a circle around the number.

Back of Left Hand   **Back of Right Hand**

Left Arm

Top of Forearm   **Bottom of Forearm**

Right Arm

Top of Forearm   **Bottom of Forearm**

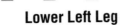

Lab

Prickle Puzzles continued

Left Upper Arm   **Right Upper Arm**   **Lower Left Leg**   **Lower Right Leg**

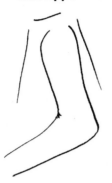 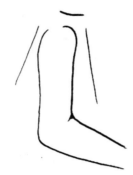   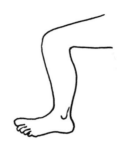 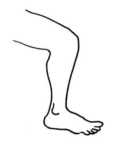

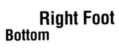

Left Foot   **Right Foot**
Top   **Bottom**   **Bottom**   **Top**

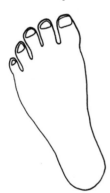 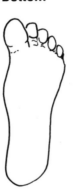   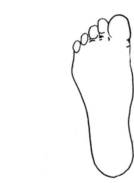 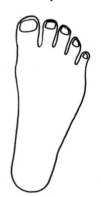

Back of Neck   **Face**

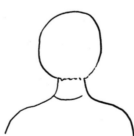 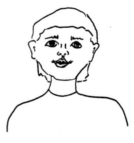

Note: Which area is the most sensitive to pressure? Why?

_____

_____

From *Bones, Bodies and Bellies*, published by GoodYearBooks. Copyright © 1994 Diane A. Vaszily and Peggy K. Perdue.

Walking the Straight and Narrow

Humans maintain balance because of muscle coordination, nervous system feedback, and sometimes visual perception. Doctors use tests like the one in this activity to determine whether a person has a spinal cord injury, is under the influence of a nerve inhibitor such as alcohol or drugs, or has muscle tone that is impaired. Students will learn that balance, even when walking, is a delicate combination of nerve impulse, muscle tone, and visual messages.

Materials

A straight line on the ground ten yards long. You may draw this line on the floor, playground, or sidewalk, or use a carpenter's chalk line (string rubbed in chalk dust, held at both ends and snapped in the middle), or place red or orange tape on the ground.

How to Do It

Have the subject stand at one end of the chalk line facing the other end. For the first test, hands should be down and next to the body, and the eyes should be open. The subject should walk straight ahead, placing one foot in front of the other. The head should be up, and the eyes should focus straight ahead.

Repeat the procedure for the second test, except extend the arms 90°.

For the third test, walk with arms at side and eyes closed.

Repeat for the fourth test, except extend the arms 90°.

Data Collecting and Recording

Use the Bodylog to record the results of the four tests. Draw a solid line to mark the path the subject walked. Repeat each test if time allows. Use a different color of pencil or marker for each trial.

Extension Activities

■ Carry out the tests after gym class or a strenuous activity. How do the results compare?

■ Try the tests at different times during the day. Are the results the same first thing in the morning as they are right before bed?

From *Bones, Bodies and Bellies*, published by GoodYearBooks. Copyright © 1994 Diane A. Vaszily and Peggy K. Perdue.

Lab

Walk a Straight Line

Balance Status Report

Practitioner note: Have the patient walk a straight line following the directions listed for each test. Draw the actual path the patient walks.

Test #1—Eyes Open Arms at Side	Test #2—Eyes Open Arms out 90°
↓	↓
Test #3—Eyes Closed Arms at Side	**Test #4—Eyes Closed Arms out 90°**
↓	↓

Note: When is the patient the most accurate? Why?

_____

_____

Try the tests more than once. Use a different marker for each trial. Can the patient learn to be more accurate? Why or why not?

_____

_____

From *Bones, Bodies and Bellies*, published by GoodYearBooks. Copyright © 1994 Diane A. Vaszily and Peggy K. Perdue.

The Great Cover-Up

Bacteria and viruses can travel rapidly through the air. We constantly tell our students to cover their mouths when they cough or sneeze. This activity provides a graphic illustration of how easily germs can spread.

Materials

Talcum powder or powdered sugar
Manual tire pump
Spoon
Tissues
Handkerchief
Tape measure or measuring stick
Newspaper
Bodylog
Pencil

How to Do It

🚫 Caution: Keep the powder away from eyes.

Place a level spoonful of powder directly in front of the end of the hose on the tire pump. Lower the pump handle one time. Observe what happens to the powder. Now place a level spoonful of powder into a folded tissue. Place the end of the hose inside the tissue and hold while the tire pump handle is lowered. Repeat using a cloth handkerchief.

Data Collecting and Recording

Use the tape measure to measure the distance the powder traveled each time the handle of the tire pump was lowered. Record this information in the Bodylog.

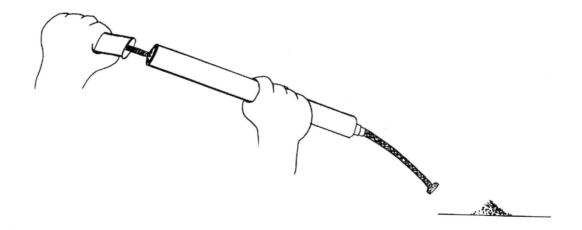

Extension Activities

■   Have students place the palms of their hands into the container of powder. Conduct class as usual—well, at least try! Have students then inspect the room for "germs" (the powder). Record the locations where the powder is found. Did the students see any airborne germs? Discuss how washing the hands might affect the results.

■   Test different brands of tissue to see which brand is the most effective in containing the "germs."

Lab Technician(s): _____

Date: _____

The Great Cover-Up

Laboratory Report Form

Lab technician note: Keep "germ powder" away from the eyes. Place a level spoonful of powder directly in front of the end of the hose on the tire pump. Lower the pump handle one time. Measure the distance the germs travel. Record your findings on the chart.

Now place a level spoonful of powder into a folded tissue. Place the end of the hose inside the tissue and hold it while the tire pump handle is lowered. Measure the distance the germs travel. Record your findings on the chart. Repeat, using a handkerchief instead of a tissue.

GERM BARRIER	DISTANCE GERMS TRAVEL
None	
Tissue	
Handkerchief	

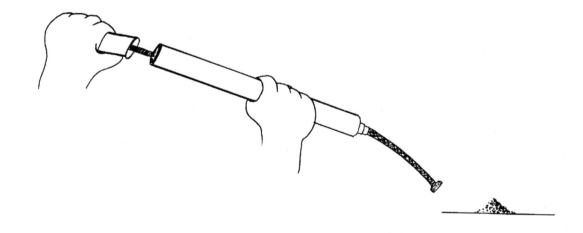

In the Blink of an Eye

Picture your room with all the students quietly at work (OK, so maybe it's not your room). Suddenly a book drops to the floor...and several students respond by jumping off their chairs. The students' reaction is an example of a reflex act. Reflexes happen quickly. They involve the nerves and spinal cord, but not the brain. Let's explore one reflex—blinking!

Materials

Clear plastic sheet
Paper
Chair
Partner
Bodylog
Pencil

How to Do It

Have one student sit in a chair and hold the clear plastic sheet approximately three inches from his or her face. A second student should wad up a piece of paper into a ball and throw it gently at the plastic. A third student should watch the first student for any reaction. Repeat the activity, but hold the plastic six inches away. Try nine, twelve, fifteen, eighteen, twenty-one, and twenty-four inches.

Data Collecting and Recording

Record reactions on the chart. Compare. Is there a difference in the reaction?

Extension Activities

- Do this activity at different times of the day. Compare the results.
- Try different colors of paper balls. Does color affect reactions?
- Try different sizes of paper balls. Does size affect reactions?
- Have students create other activities to test reflexes. Let students demonstrate their tests.
- Ask a medical practitioner to come in and demonstrate how to test reflexes using a reflex hammer.

From Bones, Bodies and Bellies, published by GoodYearBooks. Copyright © 1994 Diane A. Vaszily and Peggy K. Perdue.

Medical Record for: _____

Practitioner(s): _____ Date: _____

In the Blink of an Eye

Patient Reflex Record

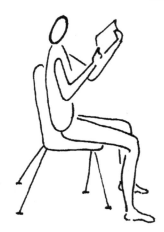

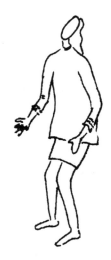

Practitioner note: You may want to get another practitioner to help you with this test. Have the patient sit in a chair and hold the clear plastic sheet approximately three inches from his or her face. Wad up a piece of paper into a ball and throw it gently at the plastic. Watch the first student for any reaction. Repeat the activity, but hold the plastic six inches away. Try nine, twelve, fifteen, eighteen, twenty-one, and twenty-four inches.

DISTANCE FROM FACE	REACTION
3 inches	
6 inches	
9 inches	
12 inches	
15 inches	
18 inches	
21 inches	
24 inches	

What's Chew with You?

Chew your food! We have heard the statement and perhaps even said it, but why is it important? Digestion starts in our mouths. Breaking food into small pieces allows digestion to occur more rapidly. This activity provides a comparison that students will readily see!

Materials

Sugar cubes (2)
Mortar and pestle, or something to crush 1 sugar cube
Clear glasses
Water
Stopwatch or clock with second hand
Bodylog
Pencil

How to Do It

Crush one of the sugar cubes into grains of sugar. Fill each glass 3/4 full of water. Drop the crushed sugar cube into one glass at the same time as you drop the whole sugar cube into the other glass. Time how long it takes the sugar to dissolve in each glass. How does this relate to chewing food thoroughly? Have students discuss their results.

Data Collecting and Recording

Students should record the time it takes the sugar to dissolve in each glass. Record the times in the Bodylog. Have teams compare their findings. Complete the chart in the Bodylog.

Extension Activities

- Have students investigate the function of each type of tooth: incisors (cutting), canine (tearing), and molars (grinding and crushing).
- Not all food begins the digestion process as quickly as sugar. Repeat the experiment with other foods, such as a carrot, a piece of beef, and a cracker. Compare how long it takes each to dissolve. Discuss the function of saliva.

From *Bones, Bodies and Bellies*, published by GoodYearBooks. Copyright © 1994 Diane A. Vaszily and Peggy K. Perdue.

Lab Technician(s): _____

Date: _____

What's Chew with You?

Laboratory Report Form

Lab technician note: Follow the procedures to conduct this laboratory investigation.

Procedure:

1. Crush one of the sugar cubes into grains of sugar.
2. Fill each glass 3/4 full of water.
3. Drop the crushed sugar cube into one glass. At the same time, drop the whole sugar cube into the other glass.
4. Time how long it takes the sugar to dissolve in each glass.

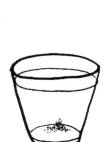
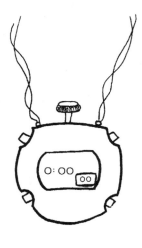
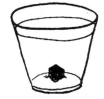

TYPE OF SUGAR	TIME TO DISSOLVE
Crushed Sugar Cube	
Whole Sugar Cube	

Compare your results with other colleagues. Are their results the same as yours? How does this relate to chewing food thoroughly?

Keep the Change!

Digestion of food begins in the mouth. Saliva begins working on food so that it can be absorbed into the bloodstream more readily. With the help of saliva, starch begins its transformation into sugar. Have students test their taste buds to see if they can detect the change.

Materials

Soda cracker
Bodylog
Pencil
Stopwatch or clock with second hand

How to Do It

Check for food allergies before beginning this activity.
Place half of a soda cracker in your mouth. Chew the cracker for 15 seconds. Don't swallow it! Move it over your tongue so that it mixes with saliva. Don't swallow for 1 minute.

Data Collecting and Recording

Record in the Bodylog how the cracker initially tastes. Record any perceived changes in texture and taste.

Extension Activities

■   Use Benedict's solution to test what changes occurred in the cracker. See "Sugar Search" on page 63 for instructions.

■   Try other types of food. Which foods change the most in the mouth?

From *Bones, Bodies and Bellies*, published by GoodYearBooks. Copyright © 1994 Diane A. Vaszily and Peggy K. Perdue.

Lab Technician(s): _____

Date: _____

Keep the Change!

Laboratory Report Form

Lab technician note: Place half of a soda cracker in your mouth. Record how the cracker feels and tastes. Chew the cracker for 15 seconds. Don't swallow it! Move it over your tongue so that it mixes with saliva. Don't swallow for at least one minute. Record how the cracker feels and tastes every 15 seconds. Try not to swallow for two minutes.

TIME	OBSERVATIONS
Start	
15 seconds	
30 seconds	
45 seconds	
1 minute	
1 min. 15 sec.	
1 min. 30 sec.	
1 min. 45 sec.	
2 minutes	

How does the cracker change? What happens in the mouth to start digestion?

_____

_____

A Little at a Time

All living organisms are made from cells. Our bodies are made from trillions of cells. Cells in the body are made up of different parts. The nucleus controls all the cell's activities. For a cell to work efficiently, it must receive energy from the foods we eat. How do cells utilize the food that we eat? In this demonstration activity, students will see how osmosis works.

Materials

Plastic sandwich bag
1/4 cup measuring cup
1/4 teaspoon measuring spoon
Eyedropper
Scissors
Iodine
Water
Cornstarch
Waxed paper
String or twist tie
Clear, plastic glass
Pencils
Paper or Bodylog

How to Do It

Make a 10 percent iodine solution (one part iodine to ten parts water).

⊘ Caution: Iodine is poisonous. Use with care. Iodine will permanently stain clothes. Have students wear protective clothing (lab coats) and rubber gloves.

Show students how iodine reacts in the presence of starch. Place a small amount of cornstarch on a piece of waxed paper. Have students observe the color of the iodine solution. Add one or two drops of the solution to the cornstarch. The iodine immediately turns purple. Iodine turns purple in the presence of starch.

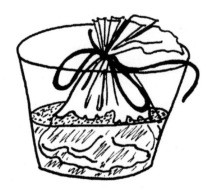

Have students make a cell model using a plastic sandwich bag. The bag represents the cell membrane. Its function is to hold the cell together. Pour 1/4 cup of water into the bag. Add 1/4 teaspoon cornstarch to the water and mix thoroughly. Have students remove all of the air inside the bag and tie it closed so that the cornstarch solution is in one corner of the bag. Fill the plastic cup 1/4 full of water. Add one or two drops of the iodine solution to the water. The water will be a golden color. Students should then place the cell model into the plastic cup.

Data Collecting and Recording

Students should draw a "Before" and "After" picture of the cell model in their Bodylogs. Encourage students to make observations at set intervals (such as every five minutes).

Extension Activities

- Study the digestive system and the absorption of food.
- Make cell models out of clay. Label all the parts.
- Compare the cell of an animal to that of a plant. How are they different? (The major difference is that a plant cell has a rigid cell wall that surrounds the cell membrane.)
- Compare the size of iodine, water, and starch molecules. Which is able to pass through the plastic bag? (iodine)

■ ■ ■ ■ ■ ■ ■ ■ ■ ■ ■ ■ ■ ■ ■ ■ ■

A Little at a Time

Laboratory Report Form

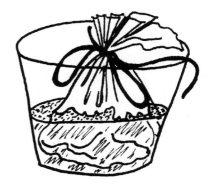

🚫 Lab Technician Caution: Iodine is poisonous. Use with care. Iodine will permanently stain clothes. Wear protective clothing (lab coats) and rubber gloves.

Follow the procedures for this lab activity.

Procedure:

1. Open the plastic bag.
2. Pour 1/4 cup of water into bag.
3. Add 1/4 teaspoon of cornstarch to the water.
4. Mix thoroughly.
5. Remove all of the air from the bag. Tie the bag closed so that the cornstarch and water solution is in one corner of the bag.
6. Cut away the unused portion of the bag, leaving about 3 cm above the tie.
7. Fill the clear plastic glass 1/4 full of water.
8. Add one or two drops of iodine to the water to turn the water gold.
9. Place the cell model in the glass.
10. Observe carefully.

Observations:

BEFORE	AFTER

Be ready to describe your findings every five minutes. Design a chart to record your observations. Of iodine, water, and starch, which has the largest molecules? The smallest?

Bellies

Nutrition

Keeping the Body Running

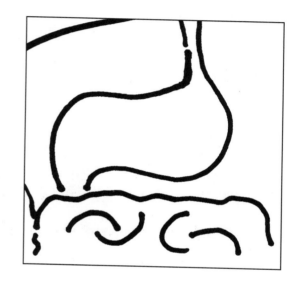

Fat Trails

Fat intake. Cholesterol production. Heart disease. These topics are in the news almost every day. Fat intake may influence cholesterol production and the resulting lipoproteins may clog arteries. To maintain a healthy diet, people of all ages need to be aware of which foods are high in fat content. This simple activity will have students testing foods for fat.

Materials

Grocery or lunch bags cut into 4" x 4" squares (enough for each team to test 20 foods)
Miscellaneous foods to test (including samples from each of the four basic food groups: fruits and vegetables, meat/protein, breads and cereals, and milk/milk products)
Bodylog
Pencil
Quadrille paper (optional, see Appendix)

How to

Choose any foods that are in a solid form at room temperature. Liquids are not suitable for this particular test. Try to provide a representative sample from each food group. Allow each group to choose its own test foods. In the case of fresh fruits and vegetables, cut the food open to expose the inside. Use this inner surface as the testing area. Lay the food on a piece of brown paper. After several minutes, a brown oily spot will appear under and around the foods containing fat. The wider the spot, the higher the level of fat.

Data Collecting and Recording

Initially, students should be concerned with only the presence or absence of fat. A spot caused by fat will not disappear. A spot caused by moisture in the food will disappear.
Try to determine which food group has more "fatty members" in it.

Extension Activities

■ Which foods contain the most fat? Cut all foods to be tested into test pieces of the same size. Put the food on the paper bag squares for five minutes. Cut out the fat circle that the food made (Be sure to label it!). Lay the circle on the quadrille paper (see Appendix). Determine how many squares the circle covers. Compare the different foods. After you place the foods in order from most fat to least fat, check the nutrition labels on the food containers. Remember that serving size varies among foods. The grams of fat may be difficult to compare.

■ Compare similar foods (such as potato chips) which claim to have little or no fat.

■ See "It's All in Black and White," page 66, and "Gram-my Awards," page 69, for related activities.

Nutritionist(s): _____

Date: _____

Fat Trails

Dietary Record Sheet

Nutritionist note: Choose any foods that are in a solid form at room temperature. Try to provide a representative sample from each food group. For fresh fruits and vegetables, cut the food open to expose the inside. Use this inner surface as the testing area. Lay the food on a piece of brown paper. After several minutes, an oily spot will appear under and around the foods containing fat. The wider the spot, the higher the level of fat.

FOOD BEING TESTED	IS FAT PRESENT?

If you were advising a patient with high cholesterol to stay away from fatty foods, which foods would you include on your list?

_____

_____

Which food group seems to be the lowest in fat?

_____

March of the Starch

Carbohydrates once had a negative connotation with regard to diet. Recently, carbohydrates have received much attention as part of a healthy food plan. Nutritionists now recommend that we consume 55 percent of our total calories in the form of carbohydrates. Because of carbohydrates' slow release of energy during digestion, long-distance runners "carbohydrate load" the night before a race. Complex carbohydrates are known as starches.

Materials

Tincture of Iodine (found at drugstores)
Water
Container to hold iodine solution
Eyedropper
Foods to test (Foods that have starch include breads, cereals, potatoes, and pasta. Be sure to also test foods with no starch.)
Waxed paper
Bodylog and pencil

How to Do It

Make a 10 percent iodine solution (one part iodine to ten parts water.

Caution: Iodine is poisonous. Use with care. Iodine will permanently stain clothes. Have students wear protective clothing (lab coats) and rubber gloves. This will add to the intrigue!

Iodine turns purple in the presence of starch. Lugol's solution can also be used to test for starch. It is a hazardous material and must be handled with care. It is available through science supply companies such as Nasco and Carolina Biological. It reacts with starch in the same manner as iodine.

Place a small amount of each food on waxed paper. Do not use paper to set food on. Iodine turns the paper purple and can give confusing results. Place one drop of the amber-colored iodine solution on the food. Be careful not to touch the tip of the eyedropper on the food.

Data Collecting and Recording

Record the reaction that occurs when the iodine is dropped on the food. Iodine changes to a black-purple in the presence of starch. Classify the foods into the four main food groups. Which food group has a lot of "starchy" members?

Extension Activities

■ See "Keep the Change!," page 50, for a related activity.
■ Create models of starches (complex carbohydrates) from Styrofoam balls and Tinker Toy® sticks or from colored gumdrops and toothpicks.
■ Invite a nutritionist to the class to discuss the role of carbohydrates in our diet.
■ Collect starch by cooking noodles to remove the starch. Analyze the water in which the noodles were cooked.

From Bones, Bodies and Bellies, published by GoodYearBooks. Copyright © 1994 Diane A. Vaszily and Peggy K. Perdue.

March of the Starch

Dietary Record Sheet

🚫 Nutritionist Caution: Iodine is poisonous. Use with care. Iodine will permanently stain clothes. Wear protective clothing (lab coats) and rubber gloves.

Place a small amount of each food on waxed paper. Do not use regular paper to set food on. Place one drop of the iodine solution on the food. Be careful not to touch the tip of the eyedropper on the food. Record the reaction that occurs when the iodine is dropped on the food. Iodine changes to a black-purple in the presence of starch.

FOOD BEING TESTED	IS STARCH PRESENT?

You have been asked to advise an athlete on choosing a meal high in carbohydrates (starch) the night before a big race. What would you recommend? Be sure to include something from each of the four basic food groups.

_____

_____

Vitamin Vittles

Vitamins make us think of alphabet soup! There are A, B, C, D, E, and K. All are essential for maintaining good health. Vitamin content in foods is difficult to quantify without sophisticated equipment. A simple test for vitamin C, however, can help students find this very important vitamin in their daily diet. It is needed for healthy bones, teeth, gums, proper growth, and strength of blood vessels. Which foods are high in vitamin C? This hands-on exploration finds out!

Materials

> Cornstarch
> Water
> Pan
> Hot plate or stove
> Spoon
> Tincture of Iodine
> Beverages to test (orange juice, soft drinks, water, apple juice, lemonade, tea, milk)
> Test tubes
> Eyedropper

How to Do It

Label the test tube with the beverage being tested. This will ease any confusion that may occur as the test tubes are compared.

Make the test solution. In a pan, combine 3 ml cornstarch to 50 ml water. Boil until the cornstarch dissolves. Allow to cool. Add 5 ml of the cooled solution to 125 ml of cold water. Add 1 drop of iodine. The solution will be blue.

Caution: Iodine is poisonous, and it will stain clothes permanently. Use with care.

Place 10 ml of the solution in a test tube. Add 25 drops of the beverage being tested.

Data Collecting and Recording

Vitamin C turns the blue solution clear. The clearer the solution, the more vitamin C the beverage contains.

Record the color of the solution before and after the beverage is added. Have one test tube that contains just the test solution. The test tube is the control. Line up the test tubes next to the control in order from the least amount of vitamin C to the most. To aid with the observation, place a plain white sheet of paper behind the test tubes. Which liquid contains the most vitamin C? Compare nutritional labels. Note that not all serving sizes are the same so comparison may be difficult.

Extension Activities

- Have students bring in other foods from home and test for vitamin C content.
- Have a nutritionist visit the classroom to talk to the children about vitamins and a balanced diet.

From *Bones, Bodies and Bellies*, published by GoodYearBooks. Copyright © 1994 Diane A. Vaszily and Peggy K. Perdue.

- Test various multivitamins with the solution. Is there a difference? Compare with a vitamin C tablet.
- Obtain labels from vitamin tablet bottles. Compare the contents.
- Place a chicken bone in a vinegar solution for several days. The resulting bone is what one would be like if sufficient vitamins were not available in the daily diet.
- Several plants may be brought to class and watered with vitamin enriched water in varying degrees. Make observations over several weeks and compare.
- See "It's All in Black and White," page 66, for a related activity.

From *Bones, Bodies and Bellies*, published by GoodYearBooks. Copyright © 1994 Diane A. Vaszily and Peggy K. Perdue.

Nutritionist(s): _____

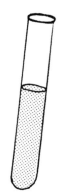

Lab

Date: _____

Vitamin Vittles

Dietary Record Sheet

Nutritionist note: Label your test tube with the name of the beverage being tested. Place 10 ml of the test solution into the test tube. Add 25 drops of the beverage being tested. Vitamin C turns the blue solution clear. The clearer the solution, the more vitamin C the beverage contains.

BEVERAGE BEING TESTED	COLOR OF SOLUTION	NUMBER DARKEST TO LIGHTEST

You have a patient that wants healthy teeth and gums. Which foods, high in vitamin C, would you recommend?

_____

_____

From *Bones, Bodies and Bellies*, published by GoodYearBooks. Copyright © 1994 Diane A. Vaszily and Peggy K. Perdue.

Sugar Search

Sugar-coated cereals, candies, and gum—all contain sugars (some are now man-made). Sugars are of questionable value, since sugar is easily stored by the body and seems to affect behavior patterns. You might want to preface this activity with a discussion of sugar and its evils as well as its assets. Simple sugars provide the fuel our body needs to maintain activity. But how much is enough? While this activity cannot answer that, it can help students identify foods that contain sugar.

Materials

Benedict's solution (commercially available through science supply companies). Glucose testing paper or Clinitest tablets may also be used. They are not as reliable, but they are acceptable. They can be found at most drug stores.
Eyedropper
Test tubes or clear bottles of the same size
Water
Hot plate or stove
Pan to heat water
Glass measuring cup or beaker to hold test tubes upright
Foods to be tested
Test tube holder
Measuring spoons
Bodylog
Pencil

How to Do It

Each piece of the food to be tested should be about the size of a grape. Mash the food. Put it in the test tube. Add one tablespoon of warm water. Shake vigorously so that any sugar that is present will be dissolved in the water. Add two droppersful of Benedict's solution to the water. (If you are using the glucose paper, dip the paper into the tube.)

Fill the pan and the glass measuring cup 1/3 to 1/2 full of water. Place the test tubes into the measuring cup. Heat the water until it is hot to the touch. The test tubes must be left in the hot water for several minutes.

Data Collecting and Recording

Benedict's solution changes color in the presence of sugar. Green indicates some sugar. Yellow-orange indicates more sugar. Bright orange to brick red indicates a high concentration of sugar.

Use the color changes to deduce whether or not sugar is present. Prepare a chart of the foods used and indicate the color of the Benedict's solution. How much sugar is in each food sample?

It's All in Black and White

Recently a leading peanut butter manufacturer began advertising a new peanut butter that contained less sugar and salt. Tempted to buy the product, I compared the nutrition label of the new product to the "old" product. The labels were almost the same. The calories, fats, and proteins were the same, as were many other entries on the list. I decided not to take a chance on the new product. More and more foods carry labels that list nutrition information. By investigating what is on a nutrition label, students can begin making informed food choices.

Materials

Food packages (ask students to bring the "empties" from home)
Bodylog
Pencil

How to Do It

Decide on one type of food to compare. Choose a food that interests your students, such as cereal, snack foods, cookies, or peanut butter. Have as many different brands of the product as possible.

Examine the labels for serving size. To compare the foods, you must be working with the same serving size. You may need to use a calculator to establish equivalent amounts. Note the calories, proteins, carbohydrates, fats, sodium, and potassium per serving.

Next, study the percentage of the U.S. Recommended Daily Allowance (U.S. RDA) each serving fulfills. What is the number one ingredient in the product? It will be the first item listed under "Ingredients."

Data Collecting and Recording

Put the products in order from the greatest to the smallest number of calories. Record the information in the Bodylog. Do the same for proteins, carbohydrates, fats, sodium, and potassium. Is there a pattern? Which brand provides the most of the U.S. RDA in vitamin A? Zinc? Thiamin?

Extension Activities

■ Is the better nutritional buy also the best economic buy? If possible, compare cost per serving.

■ Record what you eat. See "Gram-my Awards," page 69, for directions.

From *Bones, Bodies and Bellies*, published by GoodYearBooks. Copyright © 1994 Diane A. Vaszily and Peggy K. Perdue.

Nutritionist(s): _____

Date: _____

It's All in Black and White

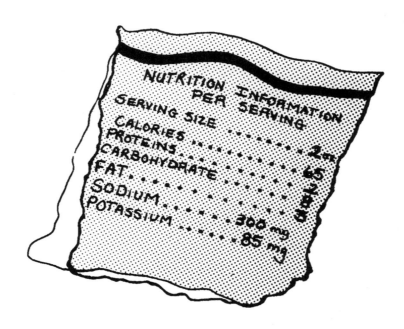

Nutritional Evaluation Record

Nutritionist note: Decide on one type of food to compare. Try to have as many different brands of the product as possible.

Examine the labels for serving size. To compare the foods, you must be working with the same serving size. Note the calories, proteins, carbohydrates, fats, sodium, and potassium per serving.

Next, study the percentage of the U.S. Recommended Daily Allowance (U.S. RDA) each serving fulfills. What is the number one ingredient in the product? It will be the first item listed under "Ingredients."

Complete a chart for each brand of product. Compare the results.

Brand of Food:	
Serving Size	
Calories	
Proteins	
Carbohydrates	
Fats	
Sodium	
Potassium	
#1 Ingredient	

Brand of Food:	
Serving Size	
Calories	
Proteins	
Carbohydrates	
Fats	
Sodium	
Potassium	
#1 Ingredient	

Brand of Food:	
Serving Size	
Calories	
Proteins	
Carbohydrates	
Fats	
Sodium	
Potassium	
#1 Ingredient	

Brand of Food:	
Serving Size	
Calories	
Proteins	
Carbohydrates	
Fats	
Sodium	
Potassium	
#1 Ingredient	

Which brand do you recommend to be the best nutritional value?

_____

_____

From *Bones, Bodies and Bellies*, published by GoodYearBooks. Copyright © 1994 Diane A. Vaszily and Peggy K. Perdue.

Gram-my Awards

Proteins, carbohydrates, fats—all are important to a well-rounded diet. How much of each do we consume? Many food packages now carry nutrition information so that we can calculate how many grams of proteins, carbohydrates, and fats we eat in a day. Use this activity to increase student awareness of what they eat.

Materials

Packaging from food, or a book detailing nutritional information for food
Bodylog
Pencil

How to Do It

For one day, have students read food packages to determine the amount of proteins, carbohydrates, and fats they eat.

Data Collecting and Recording

Have students record in their Bodylogs how many grams of protein, carbohydrates, and fat they consume at each meal and snack. When do they eat the most protein? The most carbohydrates? The most fat?

Extension Activities

■ Have students keep track of grams for one week. Is there a pattern to what they eat?

■ Invite a dietitian, nutritionist, or doctor to your classroom to explain the importance of protein, carbohydrates, and fat in a well-balanced diet. What is the recommended amount for each area?

■ Some fast-food restaurants have nutritional information posted. Secure a copy. Have students plan a low-fat breakfast, lunch, and dinner using this information.

■ Have students plan a high-carbohydrate dinner for a marathon runner.

Gram-my Awards

Food Plan Documentation

Nutritionist note: Record how many grams of proteins, carbohydrates, and fats your patient consumes at each meal and snack. Use yellow for proteins, green for carbohydrates, and red for fat.

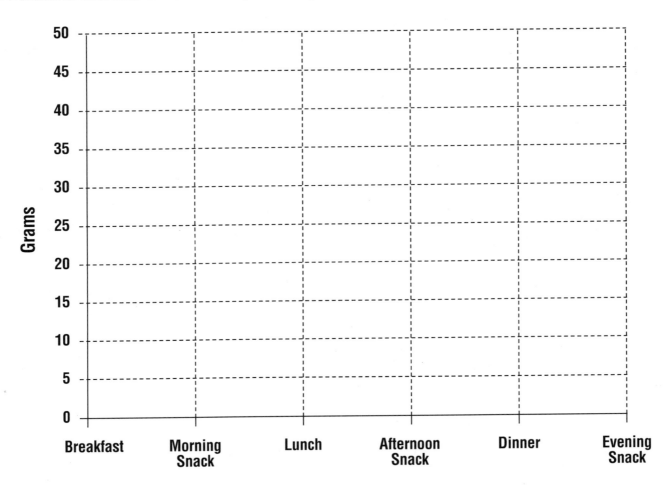

When does the patient eat the most protein? The most carbohydrates? The most fat? Keep track over several days to see if there is a pattern.

_____

_____

From *Bones, Bodies and Bellies*, published by GoodYearBooks. Copyright © 1994 Diane A. Vaszily and Peggy K. Perdue.

Every Last Drop

People should drink at least 8 eight-ounce glasses of water every day. Many of us do not drink even half of that amount. Water is vital if the body is to work efficiently. It helps to remove impurities from the body and is essential for transporting nutrients. This activity will raise your students' awareness of how much water they consume.

Materials

Sports water bottle
Water
Glass measuring cup or other container that measures in ounces
Bodylog
Pencil

How to Do It

Ask students how much water they think they drink in a day. Explain that for good health, it is important that we drink 64 ounces of water each day.

Have each child bring in a sport water bottle. Measure how much water each bottle holds. This determines how many times the water bottle should be filled during the day. Fill the bottles using full cups.

Allow the students to set the bottles on their desks and drink whenever they like. (Note: Expect more trips to the bathroom!) Refill the bottles as necessary.

Data Collecting and Recording

Students will need to keep track of how many times they fill their water bottles (otherwise they forget!). At the end of the day, they should measure any water left in the bottle. Subtract this number from the number of ounces that have been put into the bottle. The difference is the amount of water consumed (barring any spillage).

Extension Activities

■ Try this activity on different days. Include warm days, cold days, days with gym, and days without gym. Does the "kind of day" influence the results?

■ Try different types of water. Compare tap water to bottled and spring water. Add a slice of lemon to the water. Does this change the results?

■ Test the drinking water. How healthy is the water you drink?

■ See "Water, Water Everywhere," page 75, for a related activity.

Medical Record for: _____

Nutritionist(s): _____ Date: _____

Every Last Drop

Water Intake Record

Nutritionist note: For good health, it is important to drink 64 ounces of water each day.

    Measure how much water the patient's bottle holds. This determines how many times the water bottle should be filled during the day. Fill the bottle using full cups. Refill the bottles as necessary.

    Keep track of how many times the water bottle is filled. At the end of the day, measure any water left in the bottle. Subtract this number from the number of ounces that have been put into the bottle. The difference is the amount of water consumed.

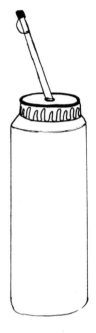

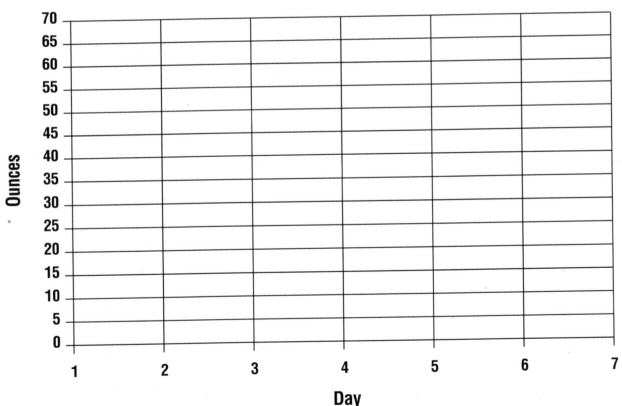

Flushing the System

Almost 75 percent of our total body weight is water! Water acts as a medium for electrolytic processes within the cells, provides a dissolving medium, and helps dilute foods. In this activity, students will discover how important water is in the digestive tract as they create a "digestive tube" for passing simulated food and water.

Materials

Flexible transparent aquarium tubing (approximately 4 feet per team—each foot of tubing equals 7 feet of intestine)
Eyedropper or pipette
Jar with tight lid for "masticating" (chewing) food
Water
Stopwatch
Paper towel
Crackers, bread, or other soft food

How to Do It

Place a small amount of food (one cracker, 1/4 bread slice, or small cookie) into the jar. Add enough water to just cover the food. Replace the lid and shake vigorously. If big chunks remain, use a spoon to simulate the crushing action of teeth. Position the "digestive tube" in gentle bends to represent the true position in the body. Using the eyedropper, draw the food up and place it into the digestive tube.

Use peristaltic motion to help the food through the tube. Peristaltic motion is the rhythmic contraction of the tube from top to bottom. Simulate this by squeezing the tube little by little. Add 5 droppers of water to the apparatus. Compare the ease with which it moves with the added water.

Data Collecting and Recording

Use a stopwatch to record start time (when food is introduced into the tube). Record the time when the food reaches the other end.

Extension Activities

■ Repeat the activity using 10 and then 20 droppers of water. Compare the times.
■ Make a solution of dyed water (to represent food) and put it in a clean tube. Add clear water by the dropperful until the food (dyed water) turns clear. How much water is needed to dilute the food?
■ See "Every Last Drop," page 71, and "Water, Water, Everywhere," page 75, for related activities.

From *Bones, Bodies and Bellies*, published by GoodYearBooks. Copyright © 1994 Diane A. Vaszily and Peggy K. Perdue.

■ ■ ■ ■ ■ ■ ■ ■ ■ ■ ■ ■ ■ ■ ■ ■

Flushing the System

Laboratory Record Form

Technician note: Place a small amount of food (one cracker, 1/4 bread slice, or small cookie) into the jar. Add enough water to just cover the food. Replace the lid and shake vigorously. If big chunks remain, use a spoon to simulate the crushing action of teeth. Position the "digestive tube" in gentle bends to represent the true position in the body. Using the eyedropper, draw the food up and place it into the digestive tube.

Use peristaltic motion (squeeze the tube little by little) to help the food through the tube. Add 5 droppers of water to the apparatus. Compare the ease with which it moves with the added water.

Use a stopwatch to record start time when food is introduced into the tube. Record the time when the food reaches the other end.

Droppers of Water	Time

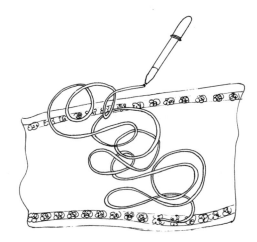

Compare your results with other colleagues.
How does the water aid in digestion?

_____

_____

_____

_____

From *Bones, Bodies and Bellies*, published by GoodYearBooks. Copyright © 1994 Diane A. Vaszily and Peggy K. Perdue.

Water, Water, Everywhere!

It's important that we drink 64 ounces of water each day. It is not necessary that all of the water come from the faucet. Water is hidden in the foods we eat. Reveal the secret in this activity!

Materials

Balance with weights
Apples
Knife
Small paper plates
Bodylog
Pencil

How to Do It

Slice the apple into eighths. Give each team a section of apple. Place the apple on paper plates. Make sure that teams have labeled the plates for easy identification. Allow the apples to sit in the open for several days. This activity works best when the humidity is low.

Data Collecting and Recording

Have students use the balance to mass their pieces of apple. Record the mass. Add each team's weight for a "Total Apple Mass." In four days, mass the apple slices again. Record the mass and calculate the difference. After three more days, mass the apple. Record the mass and calculate the difference from three days ago and from the start. Add each team's mass to compute the total apple mass. Why is there a difference from the starting mass? What happened to the water?

You may wish to have students determine what percentage of the apple was water. This is done by the following calculation:

[("Before" apple mass-"After" apple mass)/ "Before" apple mass] x 100 = Percentage of weight is water

An example is:

200 grams = "Before" apple mass
50 grams - "After" apple mass
[(200 - 50)/200] x 100 = Percent water weight
(150/200) x 100 = Percent water weight
.75 x 100 = Percent water weight
75% = Percent water weight

Extension Activities

■ See "Every Last Drop," page 71, and "Flushing the System," page 73, for related activities.

■ Repeat the activity using processed foods that have water removed, such as potato chips, dried fruits, and certain cheeses and cereals. Compare the results. Why is it important to eat five servings of fruits and vegetables each day?

■ Compare different types or sizes of apples. Are the results the same?

Laboratory Technician(s): _____

Date: _____

Water, Water, Everywhere!

Laboratory Record Form

Technician note: Place the apple section on a labeled paper plate. Use the balance to mass the apple. Record the mass.

Allow the apples to sit in the open for several days. In four days, mass the apple again. Record the mass and calculate the difference.

After three more days, mass the apple. Record the mass and calculate the difference from three days before and from the start.

Original Mass	Mass After 4 Days	Mass After 7 Days	Difference

Compare your results with your colleagues. Why is there a difference from the starting mass?

_____

_____

_____

_____

Graph Paper

Bodylog

Table of Contents

Title   **Page**

_____

_____

_____

_____

_____

_____

_____

_____

_____

_____

_____

_____

_____

_____

_____

_____

_____

_____

_____

Hand Bones

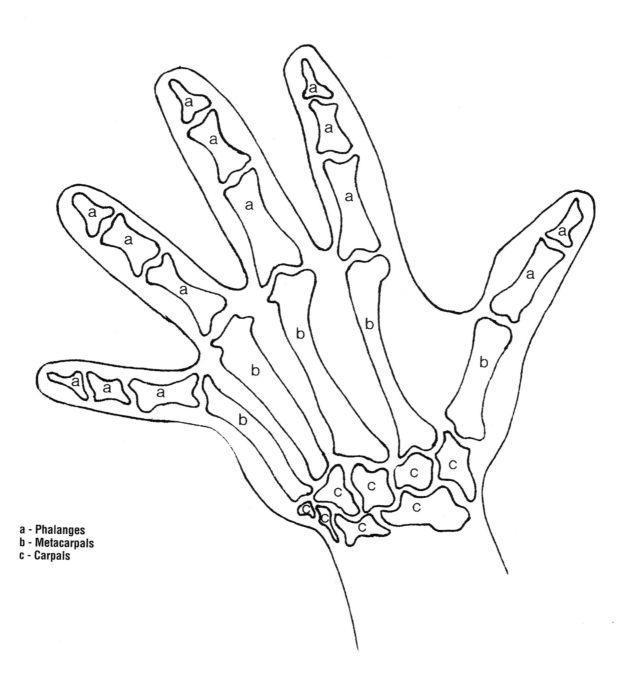

a - Phalanges
b - Metacarpals
c - Carpals

Foot Bones

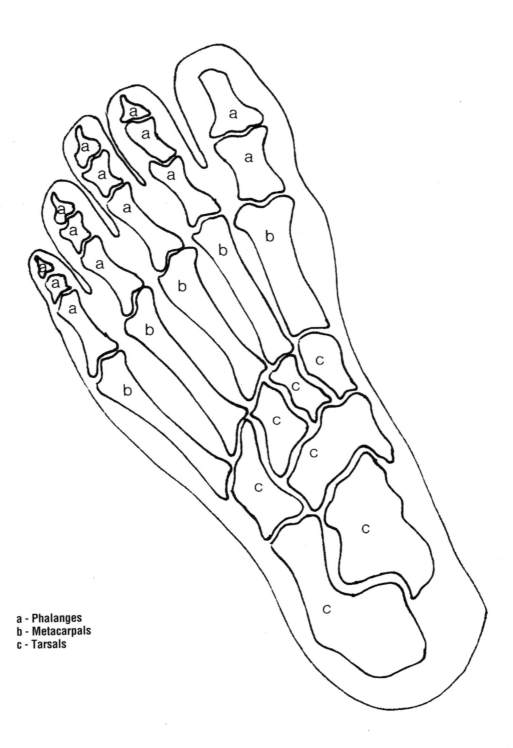

a - Phalanges
b - Metacarpals
c - Tarsals

Children's Books

Bones—Anatomy

Bailey, Donna. *All About Your Skeleton*. Steck-Vaughn, 1991.

Balestrino, Philip. *The Skeleton Inside You*. Thomas Y. Crowell, 1971

Berger, Gilda & Melvin. *The Whole World of Hands*. Houghton Mifflin, 1982.

Bishop, Pamela R. *Exploring Your Skeleton: Funny Bones and Not-So-Funny Bones*. Franklin Watts, 1991.

Broekel, Ray. *Your Skeleton and Skin*. Childrens Press, 1984.

Dineen, Jacqueline. *The Skeleton and Movement*. Silver Burdett Press, 1988.

Goode, Ruth. *Hands Up!* MacMillan, 1983.

Gross, Ruth Delov. *A Book About Your Skeleton*. Hastings House, 1979.

Iveson-Iveson, Joan. *Your Eyes*. The Bookwright Press, 1986.

Markle, Sandra. *Outside and Inside You*. Bradbury Press, 1991.

Packard, Mary. *From Head to Toes*. Julian Messner, 1985.

Parker, Steve. *Skeleton*. Alfred A. Knopf, 1988.

Parker, Steve. *The Skeleton and Movement*. Franklin Watts, 1989.

Rahn, Joan Elma. *Grocery Store Zoology: Bones and Muscles*. Atheneum, 1977.

Richardson, Joy. *What Happens When You Look?* Gareth Stevens Publishing, 1986.

Showers, Paul. *Ears Are For Hearing*. Harper & Row, 1990.

Silverstein, Dr. Alvin & Virginia. *The Story of Your Hand*. General Publishing Co., 1985.

Zim, Herbert S. *Bones*. William Morrow, 1989.

Bodies—Physiology

Adler, David A. *You Breathe In, You Breathe Out: All About Your Lungs*. Franklin Watts, 1991.

Allison, Linda. *Blood and Guts, A Working Guide to Your Own Insides*. The Yolla Bolly Press, 1976.

Asimov, Isaac. *How Do We Find Out About Germs?* Walker & Company, 1974.

Bailey, Donna. *All About Your Lungs*. Steck-Vaughn, 1991.

Bender, Lionel. *The Body*. Aladdin Books, Ltd., 1989.

Brown, Marcia. *Touch Will Tell*. Franklin Watts, 1979.

Burstein, John. *Slim Goodbody: The Inside Story*. McGraw-Hill, 1977.

Cobb, Vicki. Cells: *The Basic Structure of Life*. Franklin Watts, 1970.

Cobb, Vicki. *Inspector Bodyguard Patrols the Land of U*. Julian Messner, 1986.

Cole, Joanna. *The Magic School Bus Inside the Human Body*. Scholastic, 1989.

Donahue, Parnell, M.D., and Helen Capellaro. *Germs Make Me Sick!* Alfred A. Knopf, 1975.

Dunbar, Robert E. *The Heart and Circulatory System*. Franklin Watts, 1984.

Gaskin, John. *Breathing*. Franklin Watts, 1984.

Gaskin, John. *The Heart*. Franklin Watts, 1985.

Hindley, Judy and Colin King. *How Your Body Works*. Usborne Publishing Ltd., 1988.

Kalina, Sigmund. *Your Nerves and Their Messages*. Lothrop, Lee & Shepard, 1973.

Lambert, Mark. *The Lungs and Breathing*. Silver Burdett Press, 1988.

LeMasters, Leslie Jean. *Bacteria and Viruses*. Childrens Press, 1985.

LeMasters, Leslie Jean. *Cells and Tissues*. Childrens Press, 1985.

Parker, Steve. *The Heart and Blood*. Franklin Watts, 1989.

Parker, Steve. *Living With Heart Disease*. Franklin Watts, 1989.

Parker, Steve. *The Lungs and Breathing*. Franklin Watts, 1989.

Parker, Steve. *The Marshall Cavendish Science Project Book of the Human Body*. Templar Publishing Limited, 1988.

Patent, Dorothy Hinshaw. *Germs!* Holiday House, 1983.

Richardson, Joy. *What Happens When You Breathe?* Gareth Stevens Publishing, 1986.

Richardson, Joy. *What Happens When You Catch a Cold?* Gareth Stevens Publishing, 1986.

Richardson, Joy. *What Happens When You Touch and Feel?* Gareth Stevens Publishing, 1986.

Settel, Joanne & Nancy Baggett. *Why Does My Nose Run?* Atheneum, 1985.

Showers, Paul. *A Drop of Blood*. Harper & Row, 1967.

Showers, Paul. *How Many Teeth?* HarperCollins, 1991.

Silverstein, Dr. Alvin & Virginia. *Cells: Building Blocks of Life*. Prentice-Hall, 1989.

Silverstein, Dr. Alvin & Virginia. *Heartbeats, Your Body, Your Heart*. J. B. Lippincott, 1983.

Simon, Seymour. *Let's-Try-It-Out: Your Heart*. McGraw-Hill, 1974.

Vevers, Dr. Gwynne. *Your Body: Feeding and Digestion*. Lothrop, Lee & Shepard, 1984.

Vevers, Dr. Gwynne. *Your Body: Muscles and Movement*. Lothrop, Lee & Shepard, 1984.

Ward, Brian R. *Body Maintenance*. Franklin Watts, 1983.

Winn, Marie. *The Sick Book*. Four Winds Press, 1976.

Young, John. *Cells: Amazing Forms and Functions*. Franklin Watts, 1990.

Bellies—Nutrition

Bailey, Donna. *All About Digestion*. Steck-Vaughn, 1991.

Jones, Hettie. *How to Eat Your ABC's—A Book About Vitamins*. Four Winds Press, 1976.

LeMaster, Leslie Jean. *The New True Book—Nutrition*. Childrens Press, 1985.

Marr, John S., M.D., *The Food You Eat*. M. Evans and Company, 1973.

Nourse, Alan E. *Vitamins*. Franklin Watts, 1977.

Ontario Science Centre. *Foodworks: Over 100 Science Activities and Fascinating Facts That Explore the Magic of Food*. Addison-Wesley, 1987.

Parker, Steve. *Food and Digestion*. Franklin Watts, 1990.

Richardson, Joy. *What Happens When You Eat?* Gareth Stevens Publishing, 1986.

Seixas, Judith S. *Vitamins: What They Are What They Do*. Greenwillow Books, 1986.

Showers, Paul. *What Happens to a Hamburger?* Harper & Row, 1985.

Ward, Brian R. *Diet and Nutrition*. Franklin Watts, 1987.

Ward, Brian R. *Food and Digestion*. Franklin Watts, 1982.